LOUISE POTTER

Your essential guide to smart food choices on the go

Practical advice for eating well in any situation

This book was professionally typeset on Reedsy.
Find out more at reedsy.com

Contents

1 Introduction   1
   The concept of making smart food choices   1
   What to expect from this book   2
   How to use this book   3
2 Understanding smart food choices   4
   What do "smart" food choices look like?   4
   Why is nutrition important?   5
3 Planning ahead for success   7
   The value of planning ahead   7
   Planning ahead   7
4 Making healthy choices in different settings   10
   Eating well at work   10
   Eating well while traveling   12
   Eating well during busy days   14
   Eating well during social events   16
   Eating well as a busy parent   17
   Additional tips for healthy eating   19
5 Overcoming obstacles to healthy eating   22
   Dealing with time constraints   22
   Budget-friendly smart food choices   23
   Handling cravings and emotional eating   25
6 Staying healthy, energized, and motivated   27
   Importance of staying hydrated and nourished   27
   Tips for incorporating healthy snacks and staying energized   28
   Indulgences and "not so perfect" choices   28

Staying motivated and maintaining healthy habits   29

7   Conclusion   31

8   References   33

1

Introduction

Welcome to "Your essential guide to smart food choices on the go." This concise yet impactful book focuses on the art of maintaining a healthy and balanced diet in today's fast-paced world. Packed with quick and practical tips that you can start implementing today, this guide is tailored to help busy professionals, frequent travelers, multitasking parents, and everyday individuals navigate the challenges of making smart food choices no matter where life takes them.

The concept of making smart food choices

The concept of making smart food choices encompasses the idea that the foods you choose to consume have a significant impact on your overall health and well-being. However, it's important to note that the term "smart" does not imply a dichotomous classification of foods as either "good" or "bad." Instead, it suggests making choices that are slightly better or more aligned with your individual health goals and needs.

In our modern lifestyle, where time constraints and various responsibilities can make mindful eating challenging, understanding how to make smart food choices becomes essential. These choices should be viewed as part of a spectrum rather than being labeled as inherently good or bad. The goal is to encourage decisions that contribute to improved health and well-being without assigning moral value to specific foods.

It's crucial to avoid falling into the trap of categorizing foods as "good" or "bad," as this mindset can lead to feelings of guilt and shame. Instead, the focus should be on making informed decisions that support your health goals while acknowledging that everyone's journey is unique.

Furthermore, it's important not to judge others based on their food choices. Each person's circumstances and needs are different, and what works for one individual may not work for another. Rather than criticizing, the emphasis should be on supporting and encouraging each other in making positive changes that align with our personal health journeys.

By adopting a non-judgmental approach to food and focusing on making slightly better choices, you can develop a healthier relationship with food. This approach will empower you to make decisions that nourish your body and mind, ultimately leading to long-term improvements in overall health and well-being.

What to expect from this book

In the pages that follow, you can expect to find a wealth of practical advice, strategies, and tips to help you make informed decisions about your food choices, no matter where life takes you. We'll explore topics such as meal planning, healthy snacking, navigating restaurant menus, and making the most of your food choices in various settings. Additionally, we'll address the unique challenges faced by busy parents and offer insights to help them prioritize their well-being while caring for their families.

How to use this book

This book is designed to be a practical guide to help you make healthier food choices in various situations. Feel free to use it in a way that best suits your needs. Here are some suggestions on how to navigate through the content:

- Jump around: You don't need to read this book from cover to cover. Feel free to jump to sections that are most relevant to your current situation or interests. Whether you're looking for tips on healthy snacks for work or strategies for managing cravings, you can find the information you need without reading everything in order.
- Focus on what's important to you: If you're short on time, focus on the chapters or sections that address your immediate concerns or goals. Each section is designed to stand alone, so you can easily find the information you need without having to read everything else. (Taking this approach has resulted in some repetition within the book, as many strategies are applicable across different scenarios.)
- Take notes: Consider keeping a notebook or digital document where you can jot down key tips or ideas that resonate with you. This can help you remember and apply the information more effectively in your daily life.
- Experiment and adapt: Use this book as a starting point for making changes to your eating habits. Experiment with different strategies and tips to see what works best for you. Remember that everyone's journey to better nutrition is unique, so feel free to adapt the suggestions in this book to fit your own preferences and lifestyle.

2

Understanding smart food choices

This chapter explores the concept of smart food choices and discusses the importance of balanced nutrition and its impact on overall well-being.

What do "smart" food choices look like?

Note: Before we dive into this section, I want to reiterate that the term "smart" does not imply a dichotomous classification of foods as either "good" or "bad." Instead, it suggests making choices that are slightly better or more aligned with your individual health goals and needs. This approach encourages a non-judgmental perspective on food, focusing on making informed decisions that support your well-being.

Smart food choices are those that provide optimal nutrition while aligning with your individual dietary needs and health goals. They include foods that are rich in essential nutrients, such as vitamins, minerals, fiber, and healthy fats, while being moderate in added sugars, sodium, and unhealthy fats. These foods include:

- Fruits and vegetables: Aim to include a colorful variety of fruits and vegetables in your diet to ensure you get a wide range of vitamins, minerals, and antioxidants. "Eating the rainbow" is a helpful guideline to ensure diversity in your diet.

- Whole grains: Choose whole grains such as brown rice, quinoa, oats, and whole-grain bread over refined grains for their higher fiber and nutrient content.
- Protein sources: Include a mix of protein sources like lean meats, poultry, fish, eggs, legumes, nuts, and seeds to provide essential amino acids for muscle repair and overall health.
- Healthy fats: Incorporate sources of healthy fats like avocados, nuts, seeds, and olive oil, which are important for heart health [1] and nutrient absorption.
- Dairy or dairy alternatives: Choose dairy products or fortified dairy alternatives for calcium and vitamin D.
- Water: Stay hydrated by drinking plenty of water throughout the day. Water is essential for various bodily functions and can help curb unnecessary snacking by keeping you feeling full.

By including these elements in your diet, you can ensure that you're getting a wide range of nutrients to support your overall health and well-being.

Why is nutrition important?

Making informed food choices is key to maintaining a healthy lifestyle. While treating yourself occasionally is perfectly fine (and encouraged!), it's important to prioritize a balanced and varied diet for overall well-being. A balanced diet consists of foods from all food groups, including fruits, vegetables, whole grains, lean proteins, and healthy fats, in appropriate portions. This diverse range of nutrients supports your body's energy needs, growth, repair, and overall maintenance.

Adopting a balanced diet not only reduces the risk of chronic illnesses like heart disease, diabetes, and obesity but also has positive effects on your daily life [2,3]. A well-nourished body is more energetic, mentally sharp, and better equipped to regulate moods [4]. It also supports cognitive functions, such as memory and concentration, contributing to overall improved health [5].

By being mindful of your food choices and aiming for balance, you can proactively manage your health even in the midst of a busy schedule. Remember, every food choice is an opportunity to nourish your body and promote long-term health and well-being.

3

Planning ahead for success

This chapter highlights the importance of planning ahead to make smart food choices, especially in on-the-go situations. We'll explore practical tips for meal prepping, packing snacks, navigating restaurant menus in advance, and finding grocery stores when traveling.

The value of planning ahead

Planning ahead is a crucial strategy for maintaining a healthy diet, particularly when faced with a busy lifestyle. By taking the time to plan your meals and snacks in advance, you can ensure that you have nutritious options readily available, reducing the likelihood of making impulsive or less than ideal food choices.

Planning ahead

While it's not always feasible to plan every meal or snack in advance, taking the time to do so when possible can greatly benefit your overall health. Here are some practical tips for planning ahead:

- Meal prepping: Dedicate a specific time each week to plan and prepare meals ahead of time. Consider cooking larger batches of food that can be portioned out for multiple meals, utilizing tools like slow cookers or instant pots for easy cooking, and storing meals in convenient, grab-and-go containers.
- Packing snacks: Keep a selection of healthy snacks readily available, such as nuts, seeds, dried fruits, or pre-cut vegetables. Portion them into individual servings to make them easy to grab when you're on the move.
- Navigating restaurant menus: Before dining out, review the restaurant's menu online to identify healthier options. Look for dishes that are rich in vegetables, lean proteins, and whole grains. Consider asking for dressings or sauces on the side.
- Finding grocery stores while traveling: Prior to traveling, research grocery stores or markets near your destination. This can help you stock up on healthy snacks and ingredients for meals during your trip.

While planning ahead is beneficial, there will inevitably be times when it's not feasible. Thus, remaining flexible and adaptable is crucial, and having effective strategies for these situations can be invaluable. In such instances, it can be useful to view your food options on a spectrum, ranging from the least to the most nutritious. When faced with a spontaneous decision, take a moment to identify the "better" option on this spectrum. For example, at the airport, you might instinctively reach for a sugary soda, but pausing to consider might lead you to choose carbonated water instead. This simple shift can significantly improve your overall nutrition. Therefore, in moments when you need to make an unplanned food or beverage choice, keep this principle in mind. Ask yourself, "What does the slightly better option look like in this situation?" This simple question can guide you toward making healthier choices, even when you're on the go and haven't had time to plan ahead.

It's also really important to remember that occasional deviations from your usual eating pattern won't derail your overall progress. Focus on consistency over time rather than perfection in every meal. Practice self-compassion and avoid guilt if your choices aren't always perfect. Every healthy decision you make counts, and it's okay to indulge occasionally as long as it's balanced with healthier choices overall.

$$4$$

Making healthy choices in different settings

In various situations and environments, making healthy food choices can be challenging for a multitude of reasons. However, rather than delve into the complexities, let's focus on exploring these scenarios and discovering ways to make small, positive changes.

Eating well at work

Work can be a challenging environment for maintaining a healthy diet, but with some planning and preparation, you can make nutritious choices that support your well-being throughout the workday.

Tips for packing a healthy lunch

- Plan ahead: Take some time at the beginning of the week to plan your lunches for the coming days. This can help you avoid last-minute, less healthy options.
- Balance your meal: Aim for a balanced meal that includes lean protein (such as chicken, fish, tofu, or beans), whole grains (like quinoa, brown rice, or whole-grain bread), and plenty of vegetables.

Add in some fruit, nuts, and seeds for extra nutrients, and don't forget that the occasional treat can be part of a healthy diet too!

- Manage your portions: Be mindful of portion sizes to avoid overeating. Consider using portioned containers to help regulate your intake. But most importantly, listen to your hunger cues and eat mindfully. A good rule of thumb is to eat until 80% full (being completely stuffed would be 100% full).
- Include healthy fats: Incorporate sources of healthy fats, such as avocado, nuts, or olive oil, into your meals to help keep you satisfied.
- Drink water: Don't forget to stay hydrated! Bring a water bottle to work and aim to drink water throughout the day.

Business lunches and dinners

- Research options: If you plan to eat out for lunch, take some time to research nearby restaurants that offer healthier options. Many restaurants now provide nutritional information online or on their menus.
- Choose wisely: Look for menu items that are grilled, steamed, or roasted rather than fried. Opt for dishes that are rich in vegetables and lean protein.
- Watch portions: Restaurant portions are often quite large. Consider sharing a dish with a colleague or asking for a half portion if available. Or take the leftovers home. (And of course, pay attention to your hunger cues.)

Healthy snack options for the office

- Fresh fruit: Keep a bowl of fresh fruit on your desk for a quick and healthy snack option. Apples, bananas, and oranges are portable and require no preparation.

- Nuts and seeds: Pack a small portion of nuts or seeds for a satisfying and nutritious snack. They provide healthy fats, protein, and fiber.
- Greek yogurt: Greek yogurt is a great source of protein and can be a filling snack. Choose plain yogurt and add your own fruit or a drizzle of honey for sweetness.
- Whole-grain crackers with hummus: Whole-grain crackers paired with hummus make a satisfying and nutritious snack that provides fiber and protein.

By following these tips, you can make excellent food choices at work, whether you're preparing your lunch or eating out. Additionally, you'll have a selection of healthy snacks to keep you energized throughout the day.

Eating well while traveling

Maintaining a healthy diet while traveling can be challenging, especially with limited food options and unfamiliar environments. However, with some preparation, you can still prioritize nutritious eating during your travels.

Strategies for healthy eating at airports and train stations

- Plan ahead: Check the airport or train station's website for available dining options before your trip. Look for healthier choices such as salads, grilled protein, or whole-grain options.
- Pack snacks: Bring along healthy snacks for your journey, such as nuts, trail mix, fresh fruit, or granola bars. This can help you avoid less healthy options available at the terminal.
- Stay hydrated: Drink plenty of water to stay hydrated, especially during flights or long train rides. Avoid sugary drinks and opt for

water or unsweetened beverages.

Choosing nutritious options at hotels and restaurants

- Research restaurants: Look for restaurants near your accommodation that offer healthy menu choices. Many restaurants now provide nutritional information online, which can help you make informed decisions.
- Balance your meals: When dining out, aim for a balance of protein, healthy fats, and fiber-rich foods. Choose grilled or steamed options over fried or heavy dishes.
- Watch portions: Be mindful of portion sizes, as restaurant servings are often quite large. Consider sharing a meal or taking leftovers with you for later. And of course, don't forget to tune into your hunger and fullness cues as you enjoy your meal.

Packing snacks for road trips

- Healthy snack ideas: Pack a cooler with healthy snacks for road trips, such as cut-up vegetables and fruit, hummus, whole-grain crackers, or Greek yogurt. This can help you avoid the temptation of fast food options on the road.
- Homemade treats: Consider making your own snacks, such as homemade granola bars, protein balls, or fruit and nut mixes, to have on hand during your journey.

Finding nearby grocery stores

- Locate grocery stores: Research nearby grocery stores or markets at your destination. This can be especially useful if you have dietary restrictions or specific preferences.

- Stock up on healthy staples: Visit the grocery store to stock up on healthy staples like fresh produce, whole grains, lean proteins, and healthy snacks. Having these items on hand can make it easier to eat well during your trip. Most hotel rooms have mini-fridges in them, which means your grocery store finds can stay fresh!

By following these strategies, you can make healthier choices while traveling, whether you're navigating airports and train stations, staying in a hotel, or dining out at your destination.

Eating well during busy days

Busy days can make it challenging to prioritize healthy eating, but with some planning and preparation, you can still enjoy nutritious meals that keep you energized throughout the day.

Quick and healthy breakfast ideas

- Overnight oats: Prepare a batch of overnight oats by combining oats, milk (dairy or non-dairy), and your choice of toppings like fruit, nuts, or seeds. Store them in individual jars for a grab-and-go breakfast option.
- Smoothie packs: Prep smoothie packs with your favorite fruits and vegetables, then freeze them. In the morning, simply blend the pack with some liquid (like water, milk, or juice) for a quick and nutrient-packed breakfast.
- Whole-grain toast with nut butter: Opt for whole-grain bread topped with nut butter (like almond or peanut butter) for a simple and satisfying breakfast that provides fiber and healthy fats.

Smart choices for lunch breaks

- Salad jars: Prepare salad jars with layers of vegetables, grains (like quinoa or brown rice), and protein (such as grilled chicken or tofu). Put your dressing in a separate container. When it's time for lunch, pour in the dressing and simply shake the jar to mix everything together.
- Wrap it up: Make wraps or roll-ups with whole-grain tortillas filled with lean protein (like turkey or tuna), vegetables, and a spread (like hummus or avocado) for a portable and nutritious lunch option.
- Bento boxes: Create bento box-style lunches with compartments for different food groups, such as vegetables, fruits, protein, and whole grains. This allows for a balanced and customizable meal.

Easy and nutritious dinner options

- One-pan meals: Prepare meals that can be cooked in a single pan or pot, minimizing cleanup and time spent in the kitchen. Examples include stir-fries, skillet meals, or sheet pan dinners.
- Batch cooking: Cook large batches of meals over the weekend and portion them out for dinners throughout the week. This can include soups, stews, casseroles, or pasta dishes that can be reheated quickly.
- Slow cooker meals: Utilize a slow cooker to prepare meals in the morning that will be ready by dinnertime. This is a convenient way to have a hot meal waiting for you after a long day.

By incorporating these quick and easy meal ideas into your busy days, you can maintain a balanced and nutritious diet without sacrificing taste or convenience.

Eating well during social events

Social events and gatherings can present challenges when it comes to maintaining a healthy diet, but with some mindful choices and strategies, you can still enjoy yourself while prioritizing your well-being.

Navigating parties and gatherings

- Survey the spread: Take a look at all the food options available before you start filling your plate. This allows you to make more conscious choices and prioritize healthier options.
- Start with vegetables: Begin your meal with a serving of vegetables or a salad to help fill you up with nutrient-rich foods before moving on to other items.
- Watch portions: Be mindful of portion sizes, especially with high-calorie or indulgent foods. Enjoy smaller portions of your favorite treats while focusing on more substantial and nutritious options.

Making healthy choices at restaurants and cafés

- Review the menu: Take the time to review the menu before you go out to eat. Look for dishes that are grilled, steamed, or roasted rather than fried, and opt for meals with plenty of vegetables.
- Customization: Don't be afraid to customize your order to make it healthier. Ask for dressings or sauces on the side, request whole-grain options, or substitute healthier sides.
- Mindful eating: Practice mindful eating by savoring each bite, eating slowly, and paying attention to your body's hunger and fullness cues.

Managing alcohol and dessert

- Moderation is key: Enjoy alcoholic beverages and desserts in moderation. When drinking, limit yourself to one or two drinks, choosing lighter options like wine or spirits with soda water instead of sugary cocktails. When it comes to dessert, consider sharing with others or taking leftovers home for later. This allows you to enjoy a taste without overindulging.
- Stay hydrated: Alternate alcoholic drinks with glasses of water to stay hydrated and pace yourself. This can also help reduce the overall amount of alcohol consumed and prevent dehydration.
- Mindful choices: Be mindful of portion sizes and listen to your body's signals of hunger and fullness. Savor each bite or sip, focusing on the flavors and textures. This can help you enjoy your treats more fully and be satisfied with smaller amounts.

By applying these strategies, you can navigate social events and gatherings while still making healthy choices that align with your dietary goals and preferences.

Eating well as a busy parent

As a busy parent, finding time to prepare healthy meals for yourself and your family can be challenging. However, with some planning and strategies, you can ensure that your family enjoys nutritious meals while managing your busy schedule.

Strategies for preparing quick and nutritious meals for your family

- Meal planning: Set aside time each week to plan your meals. This can help you streamline grocery shopping and ensure that you have all the ingredients you need for quick and healthy meals.
- Batch cooking: Consider batch cooking meals in advance and storing them in the freezer. This allows you to have ready-made meals on hand for busy days when you don't have time to cook.
- One-pot meals: Opt for one-pot meals that require minimal preparation and cleanup. Examples include soups, stews, and casseroles that can be packed with vegetables and lean proteins.
- Slow cooker or Instant Pot: Utilize slow cookers or Instant Pots to prepare meals with minimal effort. These appliances allow you to set and forget your meals, making them convenient for busy days.

Prioritizing self-care and healthy eating habits

- Set realistic expectations: Understand that you may not always have the time or energy to prepare elaborate meals, and that's okay. Focus on providing nutritious meals that are achievable within your schedule.
- Involve your family: Encourage your family to participate in meal planning and preparation. This not only teaches children about healthy eating but also helps distribute the workload.
- Quick and healthy snacks: Keep a variety of healthy snacks on hand for both yourself and your family. This can include fresh fruits, vegetables with hummus, yogurt, nuts, and seeds.
- Self-care: Remember to prioritize your own well-being. Carve out time for self-care activities that help you recharge, such as exercise, meditation, or hobbies that bring you joy.

By incorporating these strategies into your routine, you can make healthy eating a manageable and enjoyable part of your busy life as a parent.

Additional tips for healthy eating

In addition to the strategies outlined in this chapter so far, here are some additional tips to help you make informed choices and maintain a healthy diet:

Reading food labels

- Check the ingredients: Pay attention to the ingredients list on packaged foods. Choose products with simple and recognizable ingredients, and be wary of items with long lists of additives or preservatives. Some common additives and preservatives to watch out for include: artificial colors (e.g., Red 40, Yellow 5), artificial flavors, artificial sweeteners (e.g., aspartame, saccharin), preservatives (e.g., BHA, BHT, sodium nitrate, sodium nitrite), and hydrogenated oils or trans fats. Opting for foods without these additives and preservatives can support a more natural and wholesome diet.
- Understand serving sizes: Take note of the serving size and the number of servings per container.
- Watch for hidden sugars: Be mindful of hidden sugars in processed foods. Look for alternative options with lower sugar. Hidden sugars can come in many forms on food labels. Some common names for hidden sugars include: high-fructose corn syrup, corn syrup, dextrose, fructose, glucose, sucrose, maltose, honey, molasses, agave nectar, and fruit juice concentrates to name a few.
- Watch the sodium content: Check the sodium content of packaged

foods. Sodium is added to foods for various reasons such as flavor enhancement, preservation, and texture and structure. While sodium is necessary for the body to function properly, excessive intake can have negative health effects. Therefore, it's important to be mindful of sodium content in foods and opt for lower-sodium options when possible.

Identifying nutritious options

- Focus on whole foods: Prioritize whole, unprocessed foods such as fruits, vegetables, whole grains, lean proteins, and healthy fats. These foods are rich in nutrients and essential for a balanced diet.
- Choose nutrient-dense foods: Opt for foods that are nutrient-dense, meaning they provide a high amount of nutrients relative to their calorie content. Examples include leafy greens, berries, nuts, seeds, and lean meats.
- Variety: Aim for a variety of foods from different food groups to ensure you get a wide range of nutrients. Incorporating a diverse range of foods can also make your meals more interesting and enjoyable.

Limiting unhealthy temptations

- Plan ahead: When possible, plan your meals and snacks in advance to avoid impulsive food choices. Having healthy options readily available can help you resist unhealthy temptations.
- Practice mindful eating: Pay attention to your hunger and fullness cues, and eat slowly to savor your food.
- Limit highly processed foods: Minimize your intake of highly processed foods that are often high in added sugars and unhealthy fats. These include items like sugary cereals, packaged snacks,

and fast food. Instead, opt for whole, minimally processed foods such as fresh fruits and vegetables, whole grains, lean proteins like chicken and fish, nuts, seeds, and legumes. Choosing these foods can provide a better balance of nutrients and support your overall health.

By incorporating these tips into your daily routine, you can make healthier choices and maintain a balanced diet that supports your overall well-being.

5

Overcoming obstacles to healthy eating

This chapter explores strategies for overcoming common obstacles to maintaining healthy eating habits, such as time constraints, budget limitations, cravings, and emotional eating. Balancing a busy schedule can make it challenging to sustain healthy eating habits. Let's delve into these common obstacles and discover effective strategies for overcoming them.

Dealing with time constraints

Time is often a limiting factor in maintaining healthy eating habits. However, with strategic planning and preparation, it's possible to overcome this challenge. Here are some strategies for efficient meal planning and preparation that fit into hectic lifestyles:

- Batch cooking: Prepare large quantities of food at once, which can then be portioned and stored for later use. This approach can save time during the week, as you can simply reheat meals instead of cooking from scratch every day. Choose recipes that can be easily scaled up and are suitable for freezing.

- Time-saving kitchen gadgets: Invest in kitchen gadgets like slow cookers, pressure cookers, and rice cookers to streamline meal preparation. These appliances require minimal hands-on time and can cook food slowly over several hours or rapidly under pressure.
- Meal preparation in advance: Set aside time to prepare meals in advance, such as on weekends or during less hectic times. This can include washing and chopping vegetables, cooking grains or proteins, and assembling ready-to-eat meals or meal components.
- Quick and easy recipes: Look for recipes that are quick and easy to prepare, requiring minimal ingredients and preparation time. Simple meals like salads, stir-fries, wraps, and sandwiches can be nutritious and convenient options for busy days.

By incorporating these strategies into your routine, you can effectively manage time constraints and maintain a healthy diet, even in the midst of a hectic schedule. Planning and preparation are key to success when it comes to healthy eating habits.

Budget-friendly smart food choices

Eating healthily on a budget can be challenging, but with the right approach, it's entirely possible. Here are some strategies to help you make smart food choices that are both nutritious and budget-friendly:

- Shopping smart: Look for sales, discounts, and bulk options to maximize your budget. Compare prices across different brands and consider purchasing store brands, which are often more affordable but offer similar quality.
- Meal planning: Create a weekly meal plan based on affordable ingredients that are in season and on sale. This can help you avoid impulse purchases and reduce food waste by only buying what you

need.

- Choosing nutritious ingredients: Focus on purchasing nutrient-dense foods that provide a lot of nutrition for their cost. Examples include whole grains, legumes, affordable fruits and vegetables, and inexpensive sources of protein.
- Cooking in bulk: Cook in bulk and freeze individual portions for later use. This can save you time and money, as you can prepare larger quantities of food at once and portion them out for future meals.
- Use leftovers creatively: Transform leftovers into new meals to avoid food waste. For example, use leftover roasted vegetables in salads or wraps, and cooked grains in grain bowls with added protein and vegetables.

Rising food prices can make healthy eating seem out of reach. The increasing cost of fresh produce and meat compared to cheaper ultra-processed foods poses a significant challenge. While this book doesn't delve into this issue in detail, it's essential to acknowledge this reality. Despite these challenges, the strategies outlined in this chapter can help you maximize your budget while maintaining a focus on health. By being strategic in your shopping, meal planning, and ingredient choices, you can still find ways to incorporate nutritious foods into your diet without overspending.

With these strategies, you can make the most of your grocery budget while still enjoying a healthy and balanced diet. By planning ahead and being creative, eating well on a budget can be both achievable and enjoyable.

Handling cravings and emotional eating

Cravings and emotional eating can present significant challenges when trying to maintain healthy eating habits. Here are some strategies to help you manage these challenges effectively:

- Mindful eating: Practice mindful eating by paying attention to your body's hunger and fullness cues. When you feel a craving, pause and ask yourself if you are truly hungry or if there is an emotional trigger behind the craving. By being mindful of your eating habits, you can avoid unnecessary snacking and make more conscious food choices.
- Stress management: Identify alternative coping mechanisms for stress that don't involve food. Engage in activities such as exercise, meditation, or hobbies that help you relax and reduce stress levels without turning to food for comfort.
- Create a supportive environment: Surround yourself with a supportive environment that encourages healthy eating habits. This can include seeking support from friends or family members who share your health goals, joining a community or online group focused on healthy living, or working with a professional such as a dietitian or therapist if needed.
- Address emotional triggers: Identify and address the emotional triggers that lead to emotional eating. This can involve keeping a journal to track your emotions and eating patterns, seeking professional help to work through underlying emotional issues, or finding healthier ways to cope with emotions such as talking to a friend or practicing relaxation techniques.
- Plan for occasional treats: Allow yourself to enjoy occasional treats in moderation. Depriving yourself completely of foods you enjoy can lead to feelings of deprivation and ultimately, binge eating.

Instead, practice portion control and savor your treats mindfully.

By implementing these strategies, you can develop a healthier relationship with food, manage cravings and emotional eating more effectively, and stay on track with your healthy eating goals.

6

Staying healthy, energized, and motivated

This chapter discusses strategies for maintaining your energy and well-being, especially during travel or busy days. It explores the importance of hydration, balanced nutrition, and mindful indulgence in sustaining your vitality. It also looks at some tips for staying motivated to maintain your healthy habits.

Importance of staying hydrated and nourished

Staying hydrated is crucial for maintaining energy levels and supporting overall health, especially when you're on the go. Water plays a vital role in regulating body temperature, aiding digestion, and transporting nutrients and oxygen throughout your body [6]. When traveling or facing a hectic schedule, it's essential to drink water regularly to prevent dehydration and support optimal functioning.

In addition to hydration, balanced nutrition is key to sustaining your energy throughout the day. A well-rounded diet that includes a mix of carbohydrates, proteins, healthy fats, vitamins, and minerals provides your body with the fuel it needs to function efficiently. Prioritizing nutrient-dense foods can help you maintain steady energy levels and support your overall well-being, even during busy times.

Tips for incorporating healthy snacks and staying energized

When you're on the go, choosing healthy snacks can help you stay energized and satisfied between meals. Opt for snacks that are rich in nutrients and easy to pack, such as fresh fruits, nuts, seeds, yogurt, whole-grain crackers, or cut-up vegetables with hummus. These snacks provide a combination of carbohydrates, proteins, and healthy fats to keep you fueled throughout the day.

Portion control and mindful eating are important aspects of snacking, especially when you're busy. Pay attention to your hunger and fullness cues, and aim to eat mindfully. By choosing nutrient-dense snacks and practicing mindful eating, you can maintain your energy levels and support your overall health, even during hectic days.

Indulgences and "not so perfect" choices

In the context of a healthy lifestyle, occasional indulgences are a normal part of enjoying food. It's okay to savor treats and enjoy less nutritious foods in moderation. The key is to approach indulgences with mindfulness and balance, rather than guilt or restriction.

When indulging, focus on savoring the flavors and enjoying the experience. Be mindful of portion sizes and listen to your body's signals of hunger and fullness. By practicing mindful indulgence, you can satisfy your cravings while maintaining a balanced approach to eating.

Staying motivated and maintaining healthy habits

Maintaining motivation is essential for sustaining healthy eating habits in the long run. Here are some strategies to help you stay motivated and maintain your healthy habits:

- Set realistic goals: Set achievable and realistic goals that are specific, measurable, attainable, relevant, and time-bound (SMART). Break down larger goals into smaller, manageable steps to track your progress more effectively.
- Track your progress: Keep track of your food intake, physical activity, and any other relevant factors using a journal or a mobile app. Tracking your progress can help you stay accountable and motivated by seeing how far you've come and identifying areas for improvement.
- Seek support: Surround yourself with a supportive network of friends, family members, or online communities who share your health and wellness goals. Having a support system can provide encouragement, accountability, and practical tips for maintaining healthy habits.
- Focus on the benefits: Remind yourself of the benefits of healthy eating, such as improved energy levels, better mood, and reduced risk of chronic diseases [1,2,3,5]. Visualize how achieving your goals will positively impact your overall well-being.
- Stay flexible: Be flexible and adaptable in your approach to healthy eating. There may be times when life gets busy or when you face unexpected challenges, and it's important to be able to adjust your plans without feeling discouraged.
- Celebrate your achievements: Celebrate your successes, no matter how small. Acknowledge and reward yourself for reaching milestones and staying committed to your healthy eating goals.

- Practice self-compassion: Remember that setbacks are a normal part of any journey. If you veer off track, be kind to yourself and focus on getting back on course rather than dwelling on any perceived failures. Treat yourself with the same kindness and understanding that you would offer a friend in a similar situation.

By implementing these strategies, you can maintain your motivation and stay on track with your healthy eating habits, even during challenging times. Remember to prioritize your well-being and make choices that support your overall health and vitality.

7

Conclusion

Congratulations on reaching the end of this journey! Armed with these key takeaways, you now have a powerful toolkit to guide your food choices in various situations. But this is just the beginning.

As you move forward, remember that each decision you make about your nutrition matters. You have the power to shape your health and well-being through informed choices and sustainable habits.

Consider how you will apply these strategies in your own life. Maybe you'll start by incorporating more fruits and vegetables into your meals, or perhaps you'll focus on mindful eating to truly savor each bite.

It's important to acknowledge that setbacks are a normal part of any journey. When you find yourself making less than optimal choices, practice self-compassion and focus on making better choices most of the time.

I want to thank you sincerely for joining me on this journey towards better nutrition. Your commitment to improving your health is commendable, and I have no doubt that you will continue to make strides towards a healthier and happier lifestyle.

Remember, this isn't just about short-term changes—it's about creating a sustainable lifestyle that supports your well-being for years to come. Keep prioritizing your health, and I wish you continued success on your path to better nutrition.

8

References

1. Kim Y, Je Y, Giovannucci EL. Association between dietary fat intake and mortality from all-causes, cardiovascular disease, and cancer: A systematic review and meta-analysis of prospective cohort studies. Clinical Nutrition. 2021 Mar 1;40(3):1060-70.

2. Jayedi A, Soltani S, Abdolshahi A, Shab-Bidar S. Healthy and unhealthy dietary patterns and the risk of chronic disease: an umbrella review of meta-analyses of prospective cohort studies. British Journal of Nutrition. 2020 Dec;124(11):1133-44.

3. Abiri B, Valizadeh M, Nasreddine L, Hosseinpanah F. Dietary determinants of healthy/unhealthy metabolic phenotype in individuals with normal weight or overweight/obesity: a systematic review. Critical Reviews in Food Science and Nutrition. 2023 Aug 29;63(22):5856-73.

4. Taylor AM, Holscher HD. A review of dietary and microbial connections to depression, anxiety, and stress. Nutritional neuroscience. 2020 Mar 3;23(3):237-50.

5. Gómez-Pinilla F. Brain foods: the effects of nutrients on brain function. Nature Reviews Neuroscience. 2008 Jul;9(7):568-78.

6. Popkin BM, D'Anci KE, Rosenberg IH. Water, hydration, and health. Nutrition Reviews. 2010 Aug 1;68(8):439-58.